I0446353

Nursing care

In

Cardiology

The complete guide

ALEXANDRE CAREWELL

Table of contents

« The heart, much more than just a pump, is the crossroads where science meets the soul and where every second can make a difference. »

INTRODUCTION

The essential role of the cardiology nurse

Cardiology, the specialised branch of medicine dedicated to the heart and its pathologies, is a constantly evolving field. With advances in technology and medical research, the management of heart conditions has evolved considerably. At the centre of this care is the cardiology nurse, an essential pillar in ensuring quality care for heart patients.

- **The patient's first contact**: It is often the nurse who the patient sees first when they arrive in a cardiology unit. Whether for a scheduled consultation, hospitalisation or cardiac emergency, the nurse is the first person to assess the patient's condition, reassure them and prepare them for the examinations or treatments to come.
- **Continuous monitoring**: Cardiology patients require constant monitoring, given the potential risks associated with their pathologies. Cardiology nurses are specifically trained to detect any signs of deterioration or complications, such as cardiac arrhythmias, heart failure or post-operative complications.
- **Managing treatment and medication**: As well as monitoring, the nurse is also responsible for administering medication, which is often vital for the heart patient. This requires in-depth knowledge of the various drugs, their interactions, appropriate dosages and possible side effects.
- **Education and advice**: A key element of recovery and prevention in cardiology is patient education.

Nurses play a crucial role in advising patients on lifestyle changes, making them aware of the importance of medication or teaching them to recognise the warning signs of a heart problem.

- **Interprofessional collaboration**: Cardiology nurses do not work alone. They work closely with cardiologists, cardiac surgeons, laboratory technicians, physiotherapists and other healthcare professionals. This collaboration ensures holistic patient care, where every aspect of the patient's care is meticulously planned and executed.
- **Emotional support**: Receiving a diagnosis of heart disease can be overwhelming. The nurse is often the main emotional support for the patient and their family, offering comfort, a listening ear and reassurance throughout the care process.

The cardiology nurse is much more than a simple performer of medical tasks. They are the vigilant guardians of heart health, the patient's confidant, the educator, the care coordinator and the essential link between the patient and the medical team. In the complex and constantly changing world of cardiology, their role is absolutely essential.

A brief introduction to cardiology : its challenges and progress

Cardiology is the branch of medicine that studies the heart, how it works and its diseases. It is also concerned with blood vessels and blood circulation. With the evolution of medical knowledge, technologies and treatments, cardiology has undergone profound changes, while at the same time facing constant challenges.

1. History of cardiology
   - Since ancient times, the heart has been recognised as a vital organ, symbolic of life itself. Over the centuries, the anatomical and functional study of the heart has evolved, leading to a better understanding of its physiology.
   - The stethoscope, invented at the beginning of the 19th century by René Laennec, marked a turning point in the diagnosis of heart disease, making it possible to listen directly to the sounds of the heart.

2. Major advances in cardiology
   - **Medical imaging**: The invention of techniques such as echocardiography, cardiac MRI and cardiac scintigraphy has revolutionised diagnosis, providing detailed images of the heart in action.
   - **Surgical interventions**: Surgical techniques have evolved from invasive procedures to less intrusive interventions, such as minimally invasive cardiac surgery or stenting.
   - **Pharmacological treatments**: The emergence of new drugs has transformed the management of heart disease, reducing mortality and improving patients' quality of life.
   - **Rhythmology**: Progress has been made in understanding and treating cardiac arrhythmias with devices such as pacemakers and implantable defibrillators.

3. Current challenges in cardiology
   - **Heart disease and lifestyle**: The increase in lifestyle-related heart disease, such as hypertension, obesity and diabetes, is a major challenge. Prevention and education are essential to reverse this trend.
   - **Inequalities in care**: Ensuring equitable access to state-of-the-art treatments, procedures and education

in heart health remains a challenge, particularly in remote or underdeveloped regions.

- **Research and development**: Although enormous progress has been made, ongoing research is needed to better understand heart disease, develop new treatments and improve existing methods.

Cardiology, while a constantly evolving medical field, faces contemporary challenges that require innovative solutions, heightened awareness and interdisciplinary collaboration. The confluence of technology, research and human determination, however, gives hope of even more remarkable advances in the future.

Chapter 1:
ANATOMY AND PHYSIOLOGY OF THE HEART

The heart: structure and function.

The heart is one of the most vital organs in the human body, acting like a pump to circulate blood throughout the circulatory system. This continuous circulation brings oxygen and nutrients to the tissues and eliminates metabolic waste products. Here's an exploration of the complex structure of the heart and its essential functions.

<u>1. Anatomy of the heart</u>
a. Cardiac chambers: The heart is divided into four main chambers:
- **Auricles**: These are the upper chambers of the heart. The right atrium receives oxygen-poor blood from the body, while the left atrium receives oxygenated blood from the lungs.
- **Ventricles**: These are the lower chambers. The right ventricle pumps blood to the lungs for oxygenation, while the left ventricle pumps it throughout the body.

b. Heart valves: These regulate the flow of blood through the heart, ensuring that it flows in one direction only. There are four main valves:
- **Tricuspid valve**: Between the right atrium and the right ventricle.
- **Pulmonary valve**: At the outlet of the right ventricle.
- **Mitral (or bicuspid) valve:** Between the left atrium and the left ventricle.
- **Aortic valve**: At the outlet of the left ventricle.

c. The myocardium: This is the thick muscular tissue of the heart which enables the heart to contract.

d. Vessels: These enter and leave the heart, allowing blood to circulate.

- **Veins**: The main veins are the vena cava (superior and inferior), which carry oxygen-poor blood back to the right atrium.
- **Arteries**: The aorta carries oxygenated blood from the left ventricle to the rest of the body, and the pulmonary arteries carry oxygen-poor blood from the right ventricle to the lungs.

2. Function of the heart

a. The heart pump: The heart works like a double pump. The right side of the heart (right atrium and right ventricle) pumps blood to the lungs, where it is oxygenated. The left side (left atrium and left ventricle) receives this oxygenated blood and pumps it throughout the body.

b. Cardiac rhythm: This is regulated by the heart's electrical conduction system. The sino-atrial node, located in the right atrium, generates electrical impulses that trigger contraction of the atria, followed by the ventricles.

c. Exchange of oxygen and nutrients : The heart ensures the circulation of blood throughout the body, allowing the exchange of oxygen, nutrients and metabolic waste products between the blood and the tissues.

In short, the heart is a complex but effective structure that ensures the body's survival by maintaining constant blood circulation. Its health and proper functioning are crucial to the life of every individual.

Major cardiac pathologies: angina pectoris, heart failure, heart attack.

The cardiovascular system is essential to an individual's survival and well-being. However, it can be affected by a variety of diseases that can compromise its functioning. Here are three of the main heart diseases, their causes, symptoms and treatments.

1. Angina pectoris (or angina)
a. Definition: Pain or discomfort felt in the chest, generally caused by a reduction in oxygen supply to the heart muscle due to obstruction or spasm of the coronary arteries.
b. Symptoms :
   • Chest pain, often described as pressure or tightness.
   • Pain may radiate to the arm, jaw, neck or back.
   • Shortness of breath.
   • Nausea, sweating.
c. Causes :
   • Atherosclerosis (narrowing of the coronary arteries due to plaque deposits).
   • Coronary spasm.
d. Treatment :
   • Vasodilator drugs such as nitroglycerin.
   • Beta-blockers or calcium channel blockers.
   • Procedures such as angioplasty to open blocked arteries.

2. Heart failure
a. Definition: A condition in which the heart is unable to pump blood efficiently enough to meet the body's needs.
b. Symptoms :
   • Shortness of breath (at rest or on exertion).
   • Fatigue.
   • Oedema (swelling) of the legs, ankles and feet.
   • Irregular heartbeat.

- Increased need to urinate at night.

c. Causes :
- Myocardial infarction.
- High blood pressure.
- Heart valve diseases.
- Cardiomyopathies (diseases of the heart muscle).

d. Treatment :
- Medications such as diuretics, beta-blockers, angiotensin-converting enzyme (ACE) inhibitors or angiotensin II receptor antagonists.
- Low-salt diet.
- Moderate exercise.
- Implantable devices or surgery for serious cases.

3. Myocardial infarction (heart attack)

a. Definition: A heart attack occurs when a segment of heart muscle no longer receives sufficient oxygen due to occlusion of a coronary artery, resulting in the death of this segment.

b. Symptoms :
- Intense pain in the centre of the chest.
- Pain radiates to the arm, jaw or back.
- Shortness of breath.
- Nausea, vomiting.
- Sweating.
- Pallor.

c. Causes :
- Atherosclerosis.
- Coronary thrombosis (blood clot in a coronary artery).
- Coronary spasm.

d. Treatment :
- Thrombolytics to dissolve clots.
- Emergency angioplasty.
- Coronary bypass.
- Medication to reduce risk factors and prevent another heart attack.

It is crucial to recognise the symptoms of these conditions as early as possible and to consult a doctor promptly. Prevention, through a healthy lifestyle and management of risk factors, remains the best approach to heart disease.

The main symptoms to recognise.

Cardiovascular disease can present a variety of symptoms, some subtle and others more obvious. Recognising these early signs is crucial because prompt intervention can mean the difference between life and death, or between a full recovery and permanent damage. Here are the main symptoms associated with heart disease to look out for:

- Chest pain (angina) :
    - May feel like pressure, tightness, burning or heaviness in the chest.
    - May be triggered by physical exertion or a stressful situation and is often relieved by rest or nitroglycerine.

- Radiating pain :
    - Pain can spread from the chest to the shoulders, arms (often the left arm), neck, jaw, back or stomach.
- Shortness of breath :
    - Difficulty breathing or a feeling of running out of air, especially when exerting yourself or lying down.
    - May be associated with heart failure or other heart conditions.
- Edema :
    - Swelling of the feet, ankles, legs or abdomen caused by a build-up of fluid, often linked to heart failure.

- Weakness :
    - A feeling of constant weakness or exhaustion that cannot be explained by overactivity or other causes.
- Palpitations :
    - Sensation that the heart is beating too fast, skipping beats or beating irregularly.
- Syncope or dizziness :
    - Loss of consciousness or feeling of dizziness, sometimes due to irregular heartbeat or other heart problems.
- Cold sweats :
    - Excessive sweating with no apparent cause, particularly if accompanied   by other cardiac symptoms.
- Nausea, vomiting or indigestion:
    - These symptoms, especially if associated with chest pain, may indicate a heart attack.
- Increased need to urinate at night:
    - A more frequent need to urinate at night may be a sign of heart failure.
- Persistent cough or wheezing:
    - A cough that produces a white or pink foam may be a sign of heart failure.

It is important to note that all these symptoms do not necessarily mean that a person has heart disease, but if they are new, unusual or worsen, it is essential to consult a healthcare professional. In addition, some people, particularly women, the elderly and diabetics, may have atypical or subtle symptoms of heart disease.

Chapter 2:
THE DAILY LIFE
OF THE CARDIOLOGY NURSE

The importance of observation and listening skills.

Observation and listening are two fundamental skills for all healthcare professionals, including those working in cardiology. These skills play an essential role in the diagnosis, treatment and overall management of the patient. Here's why they are so crucial:

1. Establishing a relationship of trust
   - **Active listening**: This gives the patient the feeling of being heard and understood. This builds trust between the carer and the patient, which is essential for open and honest communication.
   - **Careful observation**: This enables the healthcare professional to detect non-verbal signs of distress or discomfort, which may not be expressed verbally by the patient.

2. Diagnostic accuracy
   - **Gathering information**: By listening carefully to the patient's medical history, symptoms and concerns, the professional can gather essential information for making an accurate diagnosis.
   - **Detecting subtle symptoms**: Observation allows you to recognise symptoms that may go unnoticed during a physical examination, such as pallor, cyanosis (blueing of the skin) or subtle oedema.

3. Treatment planning
- **Understanding the patient's needs and preferences**: Listening helps us to understand the patient's concerns, needs and preferences, making it easier to plan a tailored, personalised treatment.
- **Assessing compliance**: By observing the patient's behaviour and listening to their feedback, the healthcare professional can assess the extent to which the patient is following and adhering to the prescribed treatment.

4. Early detection of complications
- **Continuous monitoring**: Careful observation can help detect changes in the patient's condition, enabling early intervention in the event of complications.
- **Patient feedback**: Patients may express symptoms or concerns that they would not have mentioned during the initial examination. Active listening can help to identify these problems before they become serious.

5. Patient education and awareness
- **Understanding the patient's concerns**: Active listening helps to identify areas where the patient may need more information or support.
- **Observing reactions**: By observing how a patient reacts to certain information, the healthcare professional can adapt his or her educational approach to meet the patient's specific needs.

Observing and listening are more than just communication skills. In the world of cardiology, as in other medical fields, they are essential to providing patient-centred care that is effective and tailored to each individual.

Handling emergencies.

Cardiac emergencies are among the most critical medical situations, requiring rapid, effective and well-coordinated intervention. Appropriate management of emergencies can make the difference between life and death, full recovery and permanent sequelae. Here's how these emergencies are generally dealt with:

1. Recognition and initial assessment:
a. Emergency sorting:
   • As soon as the patient arrives, a rapid assessment is carried out to determine the seriousness of the situation.
b. Vital assessment:
   • Checking vital signs (blood pressure, pulse, respiration, temperature).
   • ECG monitoring to identify abnormal heart rhythms.
c. Rapid questioning:
   • Gather information on current symptoms, medical history, medication taken and allergies.

2. Stabilisation:
a. Access routes:
   • Placement of a peripheral venous line to administer medication and fluids.

b. Oxygen therapy:
   • Supply of oxygen via a mask or nasal cannula to increase oxygen saturation.
c. Medication:
   • Administration of drugs to relieve pain, stabilise heart rhythm or dilate coronary arteries.

3. Diagnosis:
a. Electrocardiogram (ECG):

- Essential for diagnosing myocardial infarction and other rhythm disorders.

b. Blood tests:
  - Testing for cardiac markers (such as troponin) to identify damage to the heart muscle.

c. Chest X-ray:
  - May be performed to rule out other causes of chest pain, such as pneumothorax.

d. Cardiac ultrasound:
  - To assess cardiac function and identify any structural abnormalities.

4. Intervention:

a. Cardiopulmonary resuscitation (CPR):
  - In the event of cardiac arrest.

b. Defibrillation:
  - Use of a defibrillator in the event of fatal heart rhythms.

c. Angioplasty and stenting:
  - In cases of myocardial infarction, to restore blood flow in blocked arteries.

d. Surgery:
  - Such as coronary bypass surgery, in situations where several arteries are blocked or if other methods are not appropriate.

5. Monitoring and recovery:

a. Intensive care unit (ICU):
  - Patients with cardiac emergencies may be admitted to the ICU for close, continuous monitoring.

b. Medicines:
  - Medicines to prevent other cardiac events, improve heart function and treat risk factors may be prescribed.

c. Cardiac rehabilitation:
  - Supervised programme to help patients return to their previous level of activity.

6. Education and prevention:
- Patients receive information on lifestyle changes, taking medication, recognising symptoms and the need for regular monitoring.

Managing cardiac emergencies requires close collaboration between a number of specialists, including cardiologists, cardiac surgeons, specialist nurses, technicians and many others. Prompt, consistent management based on proven protocols is essential to ensure the best chance of survival and recovery for the patient.

Monitoring stabilised patients: techniques and tips.

Follow-up of patients stabilised after a cardiac event is essential to ensure full recovery, prevent further events and manage underlying risk factors. Here are some techniques and tips for effective follow-up:

1. Planning regular visits :
- **Frequency of appointments:** The frequency of follow-ups depends on the severity of the heart disease and the cardiologist's recommendations. Initial visits may be more frequent, becoming less frequent over time.

2. Medical surveillance :
- **Regular ECG checks:** To monitor any irregularities in heart rhythm.
- **Echocardiography:** This is used to monitor the function and structure of the heart.
- **Blood tests:** These are useful for monitoring lipids, blood sugar, kidney and liver function and other relevant indicators.

3. Medication management :
- **Pill organisers:** These help patients to remember their daily medication.
- **Keep a medication diary:** This can help monitor side effects or identify medicines that need adjusting.
- **Regular consultation with a pharmacist:** To review medications, discuss possible interactions and optimise drug therapy.

4. Patient education :
- **Provide written resources:** Brochures, books and other resources can help patients understand their condition.
- **Support groups:** These can provide a place to share experiences and learn from other patients.

5. Encouraging a healthy lifestyle :
- **Dietary monitoring:** Encourage consultations with a dietician to draw up a suitable diet plan.
- **Cardiac rehabilitation programmes:** These combine physical exercise, education and support to improve heart health.
- **Encourage people to stop smoking:** Offer resources and support for people who want to stop smoking.

6. Communication :
- **Open lines of communication:** Make sure the patient knows how and when to contact you if they have symptoms or concerns.
- **Use of technology:** Applications or patient portals can help with monitoring, appointment scheduling and communication.

7. Psychological assessment :
- **Mental health monitoring:** Cardiac events can have an emotional impact. Regular assessment of mood and emotional well-being is essential.

- **Referral to a psychologist or psychiatrist:** For those who need extra help managing stress, depression or anxiety.

8. Family involvement :
- **Family education:** Helping family members to understand the patient's condition and needs.
- **Involve carers:** If the patient has a carer, involve them in decisions and care plans.

Tip: It is essential to personalise the monitoring approach for each patient. Some may require more support, while others may be more independent. The secret to success lies in open communication, ongoing education and close collaboration between the patient, family and medical team.

Chapter 3:
TECHNIQUES
AND CARDIOLOGY PROCEDURES

Electrocardiogram :
direction and interpretation.

The electrocardiogram (ECG) is an essential diagnostic tool in cardiology, recording the electrical activity of the heart over a period of time. It requires specific training to perform and interpret, but here is a simplified overview to help you understand it better.

1. Performing the ECG
a. Preparing the patient :
- The patient must be comfortable, usually lying down.
- The skin is cleansed to ensure good conduction.

b. Electrode placement :
- 12 electrodes are placed on the patient's torso, arms and legs.
- These electrodes detect the electrical impulses generated by the heart.

c. Registration :
- The patient must remain still during the recording.
- The ECG traces electrical activity on graph paper or a digital screen.

2. ECG interpretation
a. Understanding waves :
- **P wave:** Represents depolarisation of the atria (contraction).
- **QRS complex:** Represents the depolarisation of the ventricles.

- **T wave:** Corresponds to the repolarisation of the ventricles (relaxation).

b. Heart rate :
- By counting the number of QRS complexes over a period of 10 seconds and multiplying by 6, we obtain the heart rate per minute.

c. Rhythm analysis :
- The regular interval between QRS complexes indicates a regular heart rhythm.
- If this is not the case, the rhythm is irregular.

d. Identification of anomalies :
- **Infarction:** May be suggested by specific ST segment elevations or depressions.
- **Ventricular hypertrophy:** Alters the shape and amplitude of the waves.
- **Rhythm disorders:** such as atrial fibrillation, ventricular tachycardia, etc.

e. PR and QT interval :
- Measurement from the start of the P wave to the start of the QRS complex (PR) and from the start of the QRS complex to the end of the T wave (QT).
- These intervals may indicate abnormalities in electrical conduction.

3. Clinical importance

The ECG can help diagnose various conditions, such as :
- Myocardial ischaemia or infarction.
- Heart rhythm disorders.
- Ventricular or atrial hypertrophy.
- Electrolyte abnormalities.
- Side effects of medicines.

4. Limitations
- Although the ECG is a valuable tool, it may not pick up intermittent abnormalities. Other tests, such as the Holter monitor (24-hour ECG), may be necessary.

- The ECG gives a snapshot. It must be interpreted in the context of the patient's symptoms and other tests.

The ECG is a fundamental element in cardiac diagnosis. Its correct performance and accurate interpretation are crucial to providing quality care to patients with cardiac pathologies. Thorough training is essential for healthcare professionals who use this tool.

Post-operative care :
after heart surgery, angioplasty, etc.

The post-intervention phase is crucial to a patient's recovery from cardiac surgery. Appropriate management can prevent complications, promote rapid recovery and ensure effective rehabilitation.

1. Post-heart surgery care (e.g. coronary bypass surgery)
a. Immediate surveillance :
- Continuous monitoring of vital signs (blood pressure, pulse, oxygen saturation).
- ECG monitoring to detect rhythm irregularities.
- Pain management.
b. Management of drains and probes :
- Monitoring and emptying thoracic drains.
- Checking the urinary catheter.
c. Early mobilisation :
- Encourage the patient to sit up, then gradually to walk.
- Breathing exercises to prevent pulmonary complications.
d. Education :
- Advice on wound hygiene.
- Pain and medication management.

2. Care after coronary angioplasty (with or without stenting)
a. Insertion point monitoring :
- Check regularly for bleeding or haematomas.
- Ensure proper compression.

b. Bed rest :
- The patient must remain lying down for a specified period, especially if the angioplasty has been performed via the femoral artery.

c. Hydration :
- Encourage the patient to drink to eliminate the contrast medium used during the procedure.

d. Education :
- Inform about signs of infection or complications.
- Explain the importance of taking anti-platelet medication.

3. Complications to watch out for
a. Cardiac complications :
- Arrhythmias.
- Ischaemia or infarction.

b. Pulmonary complications :
- Atelectasis, pneumonia, pleural effusion.

c. Complications related to the wound/incision :
- Infection.
- Bleeding.
- Haematoma.

d. Other complications :
- Renal insufficiency due to the contrast medium.
- Stroke or transient ischaemic attack (TIA).

4. Rehabilitation
a. Physiotherapy :
- Exercises to strengthen the heart muscle and improve endurance.

b. Nutrition :
- Consultation with a dietician for a suitable diet.

c. Emotional support :
- Many patients experience feelings of depression or anxiety after heart surgery. Psychological support can be beneficial.

d. Education for a healthy lifestyle :
- Encourage people to stop smoking, take regular exercise and eat a balanced diet.

Post-interventional management in cardiology is multidimensional, requiring close clinical monitoring, appropriate medical interventions, emotional support and targeted patient education. Interprofessional collaboration is key to ensuring optimal recovery.

Resuscitation techniques cardiopulmonary.

Cardiopulmonary resuscitation (CPR) is a vital technique used to save the life of a person who has stopped breathing and/or whose heart has stopped beating. Here is an overview of the steps and techniques involved in CPR, although hands-on training by professionals is essential to acquire these skills.

1. Recognising cardiac arrest

a. Rapid assessment of consciousness :
- Gently shake the person and shout to make sure they are conscious.

b. Check your breathing:
- If the person is not breathing or is breathing abnormally (such as gasps), start CPR.

2. Emergency call

a. Alert the emergency services :
- If you are alone, call the emergency services quickly before starting CPR.
- If other people are present, ask one of them to do so.

3. Resuscitation
a. Chest compression :
- Kneel down next to the person.
- Place the heel of your hand in the centre of your chest, then the other hand on top and interlace your fingers.
- Give firm, rapid compressions to a depth of at least 5 cm (for an adult) at a rate of at least 100-120 compressions per minute.

b. Ventilation (if trained to do so) :
- After 30 compressions, give 2 breaths.
- Tilt the person's head back, lift the chin, pinch the nose and ventilate by blowing air into the mouth until the chest rises.

c. Continuation :
- Continue the 30:2 cycle until help arrives, the victim resumes normal breathing or the rescuer is exhausted.

4. Defibrillation
a. Use of an automated external defibrillator (AED) :
- If an AED is available, open it and follow the voice or visual instructions.
- Apply the electrodes as indicated, make sure no-one is touching the victim, then press the shock button if the AED recommends it.

5. Post-RCP
a. If the patient regains consciousness :
- Place the patient in the lateral safety position.
- Check your breathing regularly.
- Stay with the person until help arrives.

b. If the patient does not regain consciousness :
- Continue CPR until help arrives or the responder is exhausted.

6. Skills maintenance and ongoing training

It is essential to attend regular CPR training courses to keep your skills up to date, particularly in view of the periodic updates to the recommendations.

CPR is a vital skill that can save lives in the event of cardiac arrest. It requires regular, practical training, particularly in compression and ventilation techniques, as well as the use of an AED. Recommendations may vary between organisations and regions, so it is essential to consult local guidelines and take accredited training.

Chapter 4:
MEDICINES AND CARDIAC TREATMENTS

The main classes of drugs: beta-blockers, anticoagulants, statins.

Each class of drugs has a specific action on the cardiovascular system. They play a crucial role in the treatment and prevention of cardiovascular disease. Here is a presentation of the three classes mentioned:

1. Beta-blockers
a. Mechanism of action :
- Beta-blockers inhibit beta-adrenergic receptors, which reduces the heart rate and the force of contraction of the heart, thereby reducing the myocardium's demand for oxygen.
b. Main indications :
- Hypertension.
- Angina pectoris.
- Heart failure.
- Post-myocardial infarction.
- Arrhythmias.
c. Examples of medicines:
- Atenolol.
- Bisoprolol.
- Propranolol.
- Metoprolol.
d. Common side effects :
- Fatigue.
- Bradycardia (slow heart rate).
- Drop in blood pressure when moving to a standing position.

- Trouble sleeping, nightmares.
- Cold extremities.

2. Anticoagulants
a. Mechanism of action :
- Anticoagulants prevent blood clotting by interfering with the coagulation cascade, thereby reducing the risk of blood clots forming.

b. Main indications :
- Atrial fibrillation.
- Deep vein thrombosis.
- Pulmonary embolism.
- Prevention of thrombosis after certain operations (such as heart valve replacement).

c. Examples of medicines:
- Warfarin (Coumadin).
- Heparin.
- Rivaroxaban (Xarelto).
- Apixaban (Eliquis).

d. Common side effects :
- Bleeding.
- Haematomas.
- Gastrointestinal bleeding.
- Anemia.

3. Statins
a. Mechanism of action :
- Statins inhibit an enzyme essential to the production of cholesterol by the liver, thereby reducing the level of LDL ('bad') cholesterol in the blood.

b. Main indications :
- Hypercholesterolaemia.
- Prevention of cardiovascular events in high-risk patients.

c. Examples of medicines:
- Atorvastatin (Lipitor).
- Simvastatin (Zocor).
- Rosuvastatin (Crestor).

- Pravastatin (Pravachol).

d. Common side effects :
- Muscle pain.
- Increased liver enzymes.
- Digestive disorders.
- Risk of diabetes (rare).
-

These drugs play an essential role in the treatment of cardiovascular disease. However, their administration requires careful monitoring because of their potential side effects and possible drug interactions. Effective communication between the patient, nurse and doctor is crucial to ensuring the safe and effective use of these drugs.

Administration and supervision side effects.

The administration of medicines and the monitoring of their side effects are at the heart of the cardiology nurse's role. Safe administration requires a thorough knowledge of each drug, while monitoring enables risks to the patient to be identified and mitigated.

1. Principles of safe drug administration
a. The five correct checks :
- The right patient: Always check the name and date of birth.
- The right medicine: Make sure that the medicine prescribed is the one administered.
- The right dose: Check the prescribed dose and compare it with what you actually administer.
- The right route: Oral, intravenous, subcutaneous, etc.
- The right time: Respect the prescribed interval between doses.

b. Administration technique :
  - Ensure sterility during intravenous administration.
  - Check for known contraindications or allergies.
  - Always tell the patient what you are administering.

2. Monitoring side effects
a. Common observations :
  - Take regular vital signs.
  - Watch for bleeding or haematomas, particularly with anticoagulants.
  - Check pain and discomfort levels.
  - Listen to the patient's concerns and feedback.
b. Biological tests :
  - For some medicines, regular blood tests may be necessary, for example to monitor the effectiveness of anticoagulants or to check liver function with certain statins.
c. Identification of side effects :
  - For example, beta-blockers can cause bradycardia. If the patient reports extreme fatigue or dizziness, this may indicate a heart rhythm that is too slow.
  - As mentioned above, statins can cause muscle pain.
d. Response to side effects :
  - This can range from simple monitoring to stopping the medication, changing the dose or switching to another drug. Always inform your doctor of any side effects you notice.
e. Patient education :
  - Inform patients of potential side effects so that they can recognise them and report any problems.
  - Provide written information whenever possible, so that the patient can refer to it at a later date.

The correct administration of medicines and the monitoring of side effects are essential to ensure patient safety. The nurse plays a central role in this, acting as an intermediary between doctor and patient, and ensuring that treatment is as effective and safe as possible. Open communication with the patient, education and careful observation are the keys to this mission.

The importance of patient education.

Patient education is a fundamental component of nursing care. In cardiology, where patients are often faced with lifestyle modifications, long-term medication and regular monitoring, active patient understanding and participation are essential to successful treatment.

1. Central role in prevention and management
a. Understanding the disease :
   * Informed patients have a better understanding of the nature of their condition, which helps them to accept and follow medical recommendations.
b. Self-management :
   * Educated patients are better equipped to manage their condition themselves, in particular by recognising symptoms and understanding the importance of following treatment.

2. Adherence to treatment
a. Importance of medication :
   * An informed patient understands why a drug is prescribed, its benefits, its potential side effects and the need to take it regularly.
b. Importance of medical follow-up :
   * Education can stress the importance of regular visits to the doctor or follow-up tests to monitor the progression of the disease or the effectiveness of treatment.

3. Lifestyle changes
a. Eating habits :
   * Advice on a heart-healthy diet can help reduce risk factors.

b. Exercise :
- Informed patients understand the importance of physical activity adapted to their condition.

c. Smoking cessation and alcohol moderation :
- Education highlights the dangers of certain habits and how they aggravate heart disease.

4. Reducing anxiety and boosting confidence

a. Active participation in treatment :
- Patients who understand their condition and treatment are often less anxious and feel more in control.

b. Open communication :
- Education encourages dialogue between patients and healthcare professionals, strengthening mutual trust.

5. Preparation for discharge and follow-up

a. Self-management at home :
- Education prepares patients to manage their condition once they have been discharged from hospital, emphasising the importance of daily routine, medication and any warning signs.

b. Importance of support groups :
- Patients can be informed of the existence of support groups or community resources that can help them on their journey.

Patient education is not simply the transmission of information; it is a process that empowers patients to take charge of their health, work closely with their medical team and improve their quality of life. In cardiology, given the often chronic nature of the disease, education plays a vital role in promoting healthy living and reducing readmissions and complications.

Chapter 5:
COMMUNICATION
WITH THE CARDIAC PATIENT

Announcing a diagnosis :
techniques and recommendations.

Announcing a diagnosis, particularly in the case of a serious or chronic condition, is a delicate and crucial stage in the therapeutic relationship. The way in which this information is communicated can have a lasting impact on the patient's perception of their illness, their confidence in the medical team and their ability to commit to their treatment. Here are some techniques and recommendations for this delicate stage:

1. Preparing to advertise
a. Choosing the time and place :
  • Make sure the setting is private and calm, with no distractions or interruptions.
  • The time chosen should be conducive to in-depth discussion.
b. Gather all the necessary information:
  • Be prepared to provide details of the diagnosis, prognosis and next steps.
c. Presence of support :
  • Suggest that the patient be accompanied by someone close to them for emotional support and to help them retain and understand the information.

2. Advertising technique
a. Start with an introduction:
- "I have your test results and would like to discuss them with you." This sets the tone and prepares the patient.

b. Clear and simple language :
- Avoid medical jargon. Use terms that the patient can understand, but be precise and honest.

c. Check the patient's understanding:
- Ask open-ended questions such as "What do you understand about what I've just said?

d. Review treatment options:
- Provide an overview of the next steps, possible treatments and their implications.

e. Take into account the emotional reaction:
- Be empathetic. Acknowledge the patient's emotions: "I understand that this is upsetting for you."

3. After the announcement
a. Give the patient the opportunity to ask questions:
- Make sure they have enough time to ask questions and express their concerns.

b. Provide resources:
- Offer brochures, trusted websites and other educational resources related to diagnosis.

c. Suggest a follow-up :
- Schedule another consultation to discuss the details, treatment options and answer any new questions.

d. Encourage emotional support:
- Suggest support groups, therapies or professionals specialising in emotional support for those who have been diagnosed.

4. General recommendations
a. Communication training :
- Healthcare professionals can receive specific training on how to communicate difficult news.

b. Self-care :
- Announcing a diagnosis can also be emotionally difficult for professionals. Take the time to deal with your own emotions and seek support if necessary.

Announcing a diagnosis is one of the most important and delicate responsibilities of healthcare professionals. Effective communication, marked by compassion and respect, can help establish a solid therapeutic relationship and guide the patient through the challenges ahead.

Therapeutic education: providing the keys to prevention for patients.

Therapeutic education is a patient-centred approach that aims to provide patients with the skills, knowledge and confidence to manage their disease proactively. In cardiology, where lifestyle changes play a crucial role in preventing complications and managing symptoms, therapeutic education is a cornerstone of treatment.

1. What is therapeutic education?
a. Definition :
- A structured approach to informing, educating and supporting patients about their illness, treatment and prevention.
b. Objectives:
- Improve patients' understanding of their illness.
- Reinforcing patient autonomy in day-to-day management.
- Promote better adherence to treatment.

2. Educating people about the disease
a. Understanding heart disease :
- Explanation of pathophysiology, symptoms and potential complications.

b. Associated risks :
- Information on risk factors such as hypertension, diabetes, smoking, etc.

c. Prognosis :
- Offer a realistic perspective of expectations in terms of development and treatment.

3. Promoting a healthy lifestyle

a. A balanced diet :
- Importance of a diet low in salt, saturated fats and sugars.
- Raising awareness of the benefits of the Mediterranean or DASH diets for heart health.

b. Physical exercise :
- The importance of regular activity adapted to the patient's condition.
- Provide guidelines on frequency, intensity, type and duration.

c. Avoid toxins :
- Encourage people to give up smoking.
- Educate people about moderate alcohol consumption.

d. Stress management :
- Relaxation, meditation and stress management techniques to reduce blood pressure and improve heart health.
-

4. Medication management

a. Understanding treatment :
- Explain the role of each drug, its potential side effects and its importance.

b. Adherence to treatment :
- Techniques to ensure regular intake: pillboxes, alarms, routines.

5. Self-management of symptoms

a. Recognition of symptoms :

- Educate patients about warning signs, such as breathlessness or chest pain.
b. Action to be taken :
- What to do if symptoms worsen or new symptoms appear.

6. Commitment to medical follow-up
a. Importance of appointments :
- Raise awareness of the need for regular checks and follow-up tests.
b. Keeping health diaries :
- Encourage patients to keep a diary of their symptoms, diet, exercise, etc.

Therapeutic education is a long-term investment in patients' health and well-being. By giving patients the tools they need to take charge of their heart health, we strengthen their active role in their care, with lasting benefits for their quality of life and longevity.

Taking the psychological dimension into account: managing anxiety, stress and depression.

The psychological dimension plays a crucial role in the management of patients with heart disease. Heart disease can have a profound impact on a patient's mental well-being, just as anxiety, stress and depression can influence heart health. It is therefore essential to integrate a global approach that considers mental health as an inseparable component of cardiac care.

1. The psychological impact of heart disease
a. The shock of diagnosis :
- Initial emotions such as denial, fear and uncertainty.
b. Day-to-day concerns :

- Concern about symptoms, relapse or surgery.
c. Consequences for self-image :
  - How lifestyle changes, physical limitations or scars can affect self-esteem.

2. Identifying signs and symptoms
a. Symptoms of anxiety :
  - Palpitations, excessive sweating, trembling, shortness of breath.
b. Signs of depression :
  - Persistent sadness, loss of interest, changes in appetite or weight, fatigue.
c. Chronic stress :
  - Muscle tension, headaches, irritability, insomnia.

3. Anxiety and stress management techniques
a. Relaxation techniques :
  - Deep breathing, meditation, guided visualisation.
b. Cognitive and behavioural therapies :
  - Challenge negative thoughts, develop problem-solving skills.
c. Physical activity :
  - Exercise as a means of reducing stress and improving mood.
d. Support groups :
  - Sharing experiences with other heart patients, feeling understood and supported.

4. Depression management
a. Individual therapy :
  - Work with a therapist to explore the underlying causes and develop coping strategies.
b. Medication :
  - Antidepressants and their roles, potential side effects.
c. Lifestyle interventions :
  - The importance of adequate sleep, a balanced diet and positive social relationships.

5. The importance of support
a. Family and friends:
- Their role in providing emotional support, encouragement and help with everyday tasks.

b. Healthcare professionals :
- Collaboration with cardiologists, psychologists, psychiatrists and other specialists.

c. Education and awareness :
- Help patients understand the link between heart and mental health.

6. Prevention
a. Identifying stress factors :
- Recognising triggers and implementing strategies to deal with them.

b. Wellness routine :
- Establish a daily routine that includes time for yourself, relaxation, exercise and enjoyable activities.

c. Regular monitoring :
- Regular consultations with healthcare professionals to monitor and treat symptoms.

It is clear that the psychological dimension is fundamental to the management of heart disease. Particular attention to the patient's emotional and mental state, as well as providing the necessary tools to manage stress, anxiety and depression, are essential to ensure full recovery and optimum quality of life.

Chapter 6:
ETHICAL CHALLENGES
AND PROFESSIONAL

Support at the end of life
in cardiology.

The end of life is a particularly delicate and emotional time for patients with advanced heart disease and their families. Support during this phase requires a comprehensive approach, centred on compassion, listening and respect for the patient's choices, while ensuring the best possible quality of life.

1. Recognising the signs of terminal illness
a. Clinical deterioration :
   * Recurrent episodes of heart failure, persistent dyspnoea, extreme fatigue.
b. Refractory symptoms :
   * Incessant chest pain, oedema resistant to treatment.
c. Functional changes :
   * Decline in daily activities, increased dependence on carers.

2. Communication on the end of life
a. Approach the subject :
   * When and how to introduce the discussion.
b. Informing without alienating :
   * Providing clear, realistic information while respecting the emotions of patients and their families.
c. Taking account of the patient's wishes :
   * Advance directives, living wills, etc.

3. Symptom management
a. Pain relief :
  * Use of analgesics and opioids if necessary.
b. Management of dyspnoea :
  * Oxygen therapy, medication, relaxation techniques.
c. Other symptoms :
  * Treatment of oedema, insomnia, anxiety, etc.

4. Psychological and spiritual support
a. Emotional support :
  * Psychological support for patients and their families.
b. Spiritual assistance :
  * Chaplains, spiritual advisors, rituals and religious practices.

5. Ethics and difficult decisions
a. Limitation or cessation of treatment :
  * Discussion about continuing, limiting or stopping invasive procedures, medication, etc.
b. Respecting the patient's wishes :
  * Ensuring that decisions reflect the patient's preferences and values.
c. Terminal sedation :
  * Used in cases of refractory symptoms to ensure patient comfort.

6. The role of the care team
a. Teamwork :
  * Collaboration between cardiologists, nurses, social workers, psychologists, etc.
b. Taking care of yourself :
  * Recognising and managing stress and burnout.
c. Continuing training :
  * Training in end-of-life care, ethics and communication.

7. After your death
a. Family support :
- Help with administrative formalities, psychological support.

b. Bereavement :
- Recognising the stages of grief, providing resources and support groups.

c. Commemoration :
- Honouring the patient's memory, celebrating their life.

Support at the end of life in cardiology is a complex process that requires a multi-dimensional approach. Over and above medical interventions, it involves considering the person as a whole, listening to their wishes, ensuring their comfort and supporting their family. It's a mission that is both demanding and profoundly human for the entire care team.

Teamwork:
working with doctors, nurses, etc.

In a medical environment, and specifically in cardiology, patient care is not the concern of a single person, but rather of a multidisciplinary team. This collaboration ensures comprehensive, optimal and personalised care. But working as part of a team can also bring its share of challenges. Let's look at the various aspects of this collaboration, from its advantages to its potential obstacles.

1. Key players in the team
a. Doctors :
- Cardiologists, cardiac surgeons, general practitioners.

b. Nurses :
- Nurses specialising in cardiology, clinical nurses.

c. Care assistants :
  * Their role in basic care and day-to-day assistance.
d. Other professionals :
  * Dieticians, physiotherapists, psychologists, social workers, imaging technicians, etc.

2. The benefits of collaboration
a. Comprehensive care :
  * A 360° view of the patient's needs.
b. Diversity of skills :
  * Each member brings specific expertise.
c. Enriching exchanges :
  * Opportunity to discuss cases, learn and adapt.
d. Continuity of care :
  * Ensuring a smooth transition between the different stages of treatment.

3. The challenges of collaboration
a. Communication :
  * The importance of establishing clear communication channels.
b. Respect for skills :
  * Valuing and recognising everyone's role.
c. Conflict management :
  * Techniques for defusing and resolving disagreements.
d. Coordination :
  * Ensure effective coordination between the various players.

4. Techniques and tools for effective collaboration
a. Regular team meetings :
  * Time for exchanges, fine-tuning and discussion of complex cases.
b. Technological tools :
  * Shared information systems, electronic files, communication applications.

c. Inter-professional training :
- Joint training to improve mutual understanding of roles.

5. The pivotal role of the nurse
a. Mediator :
- Facilitates communication between the patient and the medical team.
b. Coordinator :
- Organising and ensuring the implementation of the care plan.
c. Educator :
- Sharing information, training carers and patients.

6. The importance of mutual recognition
a. Role enhancement :
- Recognise the importance of each team member.
b. Regular feedback :
- Discuss successes, challenges and areas for improvement.
c. Celebrating success :
- Moments to celebrate successes and strengthen team cohesion.

Teamwork is fundamental to cardiology. It ensures holistic patient care, combining medical expertise, nursing care, psychological support and much more. For this collaboration to be successful, it requires mutual communication, respect, training and recognition.

Stress management and workload.

Working in cardiology is often synonymous with long and irregular working hours, increased responsibility and a heavy emotional burden. Nurses, in particular, are on the front line, managing emergencies, establishing contact with patients and carrying out a multitude of tasks. In this context, managing stress and workload is essential to maintaining optimal mental and physical health and providing quality care.

1. Understanding the sources of stress
a. External factors :
  • The hectic pace of work, emergencies, lack of resources and so on.
b. Internal factors :
  • Desire for perfection, fear of failure, self-imposed pressure, etc.
c. Emotional charge :
  • Confronting illness, death and the distress of patients and their families.

2. Symptoms of stress
a. Physics :
  • Fatigue, headaches, sleep problems, etc.
b. Mental :
  • Irritability, anxiety, depression, loss of concentration.
c. Behavioural :
  • Procrastination, isolation, over-consumption of alcohol or food, etc.

3. Workload management strategies
a. Planning and organisation :
  • Setting priorities, managing time, using planning tools.
b. Delegation :
  • Recognise tasks that can be assigned to others.
c. Continuing training :
  • Acquire new skills to manage tasks effectively.
d. Taking breaks :
  • The importance of taking time out to recharge your batteries.

4. Stress management techniques
a. Deep breathing and meditation :
- Techniques for refocusing and managing anxiety.

b. Physical exercise :
- Release of endorphins, muscle relaxation.

c. Social connection :
- Talk about your feelings, seek support from colleagues, friends and family.

d. Leisure and pleasurable activities :
- Recharge your batteries outside the workplace.

5. The importance of supervision and professional support
a. Regular supervision :
- Dedicated areas for discussing challenges, emotions and strategies.

b. Psychological support services :
- Access to professionals to deal with stress, burn-out, etc.

6. Prevention as the key
a. Recognise your limits :
- Know when to take a break or ask for help.

b. Self-care :
- Establish healthy routines, get enough sleep and eat well.

c. Awareness-raising and training in the workplace :
- Workshops and information sessions on stress management for staff.

7. Additional resources
a. Books, podcasts, applications :
- Tools for learning new stress management techniques.

b. Support groups :
- Spaces to share experiences and advice.

Managing stress and workload is paramount for cardiology professionals. By recognising sources of stress, implementing coping strategies and seeking appropriate support, it is possible to navigate this demanding field while maintaining well-being and providing excellent patient care.

Chapter 7:
CONTINUING EDUCATION AND OUTLOOK FOR THE FUTURE

Possible specialisations: rhythmology, cardiac surgery.

The field of cardiology is vast and continues to evolve with technological and scientific advances. For nurses with a passion for this field, there are a number of specialisations that allow them to focus on specific sub-fields and deepen their skills. In this chapter, we will explore two key specialisations: rhythmology and cardiac surgery.

1. Rhythmology
a. Introduction :
   • What is rhythmology? An overview of this sub-specialty.
b. Cardiac rhythm disorders :
   • Arrhythmias, atrial fibrillation, tachycardia, bradycardia, etc.
c. Rhythmology procedures :
   • Catheter ablation, pacemaker implantation, cardiac defibrillators.
d. Role of the rhythmology nurse :
   • Preparing patients for procedures, post-intervention monitoring, patient education on implantable devices, long-term follow-up.
e. Training and skills required :
   • Specific courses, certifications and additional training.

2. Cardiac Surgery
a. Introduction :
   • Overview of cardiac surgery and its importance.

b. Types of surgery :
- Coronary bypass, valve surgery, heart transplant, aortic surgery, etc.

c. The pre-operative period :
- The role of the nurse in patient preparation, preoperative assessment and patient education.

d. The post-operative period :
- Monitoring vital signs, pain management, wound care, potential complications.

e. Cardiac rehabilitation :
- Rehabilitation programme, patient education, encouraging physical activity.

f. Training and skills required :
- Specialisation in cardiac intensive care, internships in cardiac surgery, specific certifications.

3. Specialisation challenges and rewards

a. Training commitments :
- Need for ongoing training and scientific monitoring.

b. Emotional management :
- Confronting high-intensity situations, providing emotional support for patients and families.

c. Professional awards :
- Satisfaction in saving lives, recognition of specialist role, opportunity for professional development.

4. Future prospects

a. Technological advances :
- New devices, less invasive surgical techniques.

b. Research and clinical developments :
- Involvement in clinical studies, adapting to new guidelines and recommendations.

c. Career opportunities :
- Leadership positions, teaching, research.

Rhythmology and cardiac surgery are two exciting specialisations in cardiology that offer nurses the opportunity to deepen their knowledge, develop specialist skills and make a significant impact on patients' lives. These specialisations require a commitment to training and practice, but also offer immense professional and personal rewards.

The importance of regularly updating knowledge.

Medicine is a constantly evolving field. New discoveries are made every day, advanced technologies emerge, and protocols and guidelines regularly change in line with new evidence. In cardiology, in particular, advances can transform patients' lives, so regularly updating knowledge is crucial for all healthcare professionals, including nurses.

1. A constantly changing medical world
a. New discoveries :
- The impact of research and clinical trials on our understanding of heart disease and its treatment.
b. Technological advances :
- The emergence of more sophisticated equipment and techniques for diagnosing, treating and monitoring cardiac patients.
c. Changing protocols :
- Changes to clinical guidelines based on new evidence.

2. Implications for the cardiology nurse
a. Better care for patients :
- Application of the latest methods and techniques to improve patient outcomes.
b. Professional liability :
- Ethical and legal obligation to provide care based on the best available evidence.

c. Patient safety :
- Reducing medical errors and complications by keeping abreast of best practice.

3. Means of updating
a. Continuing education :
- Courses, seminars and workshops organised by professional or academic institutions.

b. Professional publications :
- Medical journals, articles, specialist newsletters.

c. Conferences and congresses :
- Participation in national and international events to hear from experts and exchange views with peers.

d. Professional networks :
- Nursing groups, professional associations, online platforms for sharing knowledge and experience.

4. Updating challenges
a. Rapid evolution :
- Difficulty keeping up with new information.

b. Discerning information :
- Assessing the quality and relevance of new information.

c. Time and costs :
- Finding the time and resources for ongoing training.

5. Impact on the quarry
a. Professional recognition :
- Increased credibility and respect from peers and superiors.

b. Career development :
- Opportunities for promotion or specialisation thanks to up-to-date expertise.

c. Personal satisfaction :
- A sense of achievement in providing the best possible care.

Regular updating of knowledge is not only an obligation for cardiology nurses, it is a necessity to ensure the quality and safety of patient care. It requires dedication, curiosity and a commitment to professional excellence.

Innovations in cardiology : the care of tomorrow.

Cardiology, like many medical fields, is constantly evolving, driven by technological advances, scientific discoveries and the need to respond to growing clinical challenges. These innovations are transforming the way patients are diagnosed, treated and monitored. In this chapter, we explore some of the most recent and promising innovations that are shaping the future of cardiac care.

1. Advanced diagnostic technologies
a. 3D cardiac imaging :
  • Provides a detailed view of the heart, improving diagnostic accuracy.
b. Positron emission tomography (PET) :
  • To assess the health of the heart muscle and detect abnormalities.
c. Wearables and telemedicine :
  • Continuous remote monitoring of patients, early detection of anomalies.

2. Minimally invasive and robotic procedures
a. Robotic-assisted surgery :
  • Greater precision, reduced recovery time, minimal scarring.
b. Catheter procedures :
  • Treatment of valvulopathy without open-heart surgery.
c. Bioresorbable implants :
  • Stents that dissolve over time, reducing long-term complications.

3. Gene and cell therapies
a. Cardiac regeneration :
- Using stem cells to repair damaged heart tissue.

b. Genetic targeting :
- Genetic therapies to treat specific conditions.

4. Augmented reality and virtual reality
a. Training and education :
- Using VR to train healthcare professionals in complex procedures.

b. Help with surgery :
- 3D visualisation during operations for greater precision.

5. Artificial intelligence and data analysis
a. Disease prediction :
- Data analysis to identify patients at risk.

b. Diagnostic assistance :
- AI systems to detect anomalies in ECGs, images, etc.

c. Treatment management :
- AI to tailor treatments to individual needs.

6. New drugs and therapies
a. Targeted drugs :
- Therapies based on molecular biology for more effective treatments and fewer side effects.

b. Immunotherapy :
- Using the immune system to treat certain heart diseases.

7. The challenges of innovation
a. Access and cost :
- Ensuring equitable access to new technologies.

b. Training and adaptation :
- Need to train healthcare professionals in new techniques.

c. Ethics and regulation :
- Navigating the ethical issues raised by advances such as genetic manipulation.

The future of cardiology is bright, with many promising innovations under development. These advances offer the hope of significant improvements in the management of cardiac patients, but they also require ongoing reflection and training if they are to be integrated ethically and effectively into routine care.

Chapter 8:
WELL-BEING AND
PATIENT SELF-MANAGEMENT

Encouraging adapted physical activity

Physical activity plays a crucial role in the prevention and management of heart disease. It can help improve heart function, reduce risk factors such as obesity, high blood pressure and high cholesterol, and build overall endurance and strength. However, for people with heart conditions or who are at risk, it is essential that physical activity is tailored to their individual needs and abilities.

1. Initial assessment
a. Medical assessment :
   • Identify underlying medical conditions.
   • Assess your current level of fitness.
b. Listening to the patient's concerns :
   • Understanding patients' fears and apprehensions about physical activity.
   • Identify barriers to physical activity, whether physical, emotional or logistical.

2. Creating a physical activity plan
a. Definition of objectives :
   • Setting realistic goals based on the patient's needs and abilities.
b. Selection of activities :
   • Encourage low-impact activities to start with, such as walking or swimming.
   • Suggest activities that the patient enjoys and that are likely to be maintained over the long term.

3. Monitoring and adjustment
a. Regular monitoring :
- Assess the patient's progress.
- Ensuring that activities are carried out safely.

b. Plan adjustment :
- Gradually increase the intensity or duration of the activity.
- Introduce new activities to avoid monotony.

4. Integrating physical activity into daily life
a. Practical advice :
- Encourage patients to use simple means to increase their activity, such as taking the stairs or walking to run errands.

b. Support groups and community activities :
- Suggest joining walking groups or adapted exercise classes to benefit from social support.

5. Education and awareness
a. The importance of physical activity :
- Explain the benefits for heart and overall health.
- Highlight potential improvements in quality of life.

b. Recognising warning signs :
- Educate patients about the symptoms to watch out for during physical activity, such as unusual chest pain, excessive breathlessness or dizziness.

c. Necessary precautions :
- Point out the importance of warming up and stretching before and after the activity.
- Discuss the importance of hydration and proper nutrition.

Encouraging appropriate physical activity is an essential step in the management of cardiac patients. By providing appropriate education, establishing personalised activity plans and offering ongoing support, nurses can play a central role in promoting an active and healthy lifestyle for their patients.

Cardiosalutary diet and nutrition

Nutrition plays a central role in the prevention and management of cardiovascular disease. Adopting a cardio-healthy diet is an essential strategy for maintaining a healthy heart, controlling risk factors and improving overall quality of life.

1. Basic principles of a cardio-healthy diet
a. Limit saturated and trans fats :
  • Understand the origin of these fats (fatty meats, full-fat dairy products, fried foods, certain bakery products, etc.).
  • Consequences of excessive consumption on cholesterol and heart disease.
b. Increased consumption of unsaturated fats :
  • Advantages of monounsaturated and polyunsaturated fats.
  • Main sources: olive oil, canola oil, nuts, oily fish, seeds.
c. Reducing sodium consumption :
  • The consequences of excess sodium on blood pressure.
  • Learn to read labels and opt for low-sodium products.
d. Consumption of dietary fibre :
  • Benefits of soluble and insoluble fibre for heart health.
  • Sources of fibre: vegetables, fruit, whole grains, pulses.

2. The key foods in a cardio-healthy diet
a. Fish rich in omega-3 :
  • Benefits of omega-3 fatty acids.
  • Recommendations for eating fish such as salmon, mackerel and sardines.
b. Whole grains :
  • The importance of whole grains for heart health.
  • Differences between whole grains and refined grains.

c. Vegetables and fruit :
- Antioxidants, vitamins and minerals that promote a healthy heart.
- The diversity of vegetables and fruit for a balanced diet.

d. Nuts and pulses :
- Benefits of nuts and legumes for heart health.
- Advice on how to integrate them into everyday life.

3. Weight management and heart health
a. The importance of a healthy weight :
- Understand the relationship between body weight, blood pressure and cholesterol.
- Risks associated with obesity or being overweight.

b. Strategies for weight loss :
- The importance of a balanced approach combining a healthy diet and physical activity.
- Avoid yo-yo dieting and quick fixes.

4. Education and awareness
a. The importance of nutrition for heart health :
- Linking diet to risks and benefits for the heart.

b. Demystifying popular regimes :
- Analysis of fad diets and their potential impact on heart health.

c. Cooking at home :
- Encourage the preparation of home-cooked meals as a way of controlling ingredients and portions.
- Suggest heart-healthy recipes.

A heart-healthy diet is a pillar of heart health. Nurses play a key role in educating patients about good eating habits, guiding them towards healthy choices that will support a healthy heart throughout their lives.

Smoking and alcohol management and other risk factors

Smoking, excessive alcohol consumption and other risky behaviours are among the main factors contributing to cardiovascular disease. Managing these factors is crucial to preventing the onset or progression of heart disease. Nurses play a crucial role in educating, advising and supporting patients in their efforts to change these behaviours.

1. Smoking
a. Effects of smoking on the heart :
   * Impact on blood pressure, heart rate and vascular health.
   * The relationship between smoking and atherosclerosis.

b. Tips on quitting smoking :
   * Behavioural and medication strategies.
   * Psychological support and self-help groups.
c. Electronic cigarettes :
   * Analyse current data on its safety and efficacy as a smoking cessation aid.
   * Understand the potential risks associated with its use.

2. Alcohol consumption
a. Impact of alcohol on the heart :
   * The effects of moderate versus excessive consumption.
   * Risks associated with chronic alcohol consumption, such as alcoholic cardiomyopathy.
b. Tips for moderate consumption :
   * Define moderate consumption.
   * Strategies to reduce consumption.
c. Recognising and treating alcohol dependence :

- Withdrawal symptoms and implications for heart health.
- Resources available for care.

3. Other risk factors
a. Stress :
- Understanding the relationship between chronic stress and heart disease.
- Stress management techniques, such as meditation, relaxation and exercise.

b. Recreational drugs :
- The risks associated with the use of drugs such as cocaine or amphetamines on heart health.
- Advice and resources for those looking to quit.

c. Diabetes :
- The relationship between diabetes, insulin resistance and heart disease.
- Strategies for managing and preventing diabetes.

4. Education and awareness
a. Understanding modifiable risk factors :
- Education on risk behaviour and its direct and indirect consequences on heart health.

b. Promoting a healthy lifestyle :
- Encourage a balanced diet, regular physical activity and stress management.

c. Access to resources and support :
- Provide information on support groups, therapies and other resources to help patients manage their risk factors.

Managing risk factors, including smoking, alcohol and other risky behaviours, is key to preventing heart disease. Nurses, through their unique position in the patient care pathway, can offer valuable advice, education and ongoing support to help patients adopt and maintain a healthy lifestyle.

Chapter 9:
GLOBAL HEALTH AND CARDIOLOGY

Comparison of cardiac practices in different countries

The management of heart disease varies around the world, influenced by factors such as technological development, economic resources, public health priorities, culture, education and existing healthcare systems. This comparison provides a global perspective on the divergent approaches to cardiology.

1. United States
a. Technological advances :
  * The rapid adoption of cutting-edge technologies in diagnosis and treatment.
b. Health system :
  * Mostly privatised, with high costs but rapid response.
c. Prevalence and prevention :
  * Epidemics of obesity and diabetes, but with a strong awareness of prevention.

2. Europe (taking into account the diversity of countries)
a. Universal health services :
  * Access to quality healthcare in many countries thanks to universal health cover.
b. Focus on prevention :
  * Public health initiatives, such as reducing smoking.
c. Research and collaboration :
  * Cross-border collaboration on research and clinical studies.
3. Africa
a. Limited access to care :

- In many countries, resources for cardiology are limited.
b. Emerging diseases :
  - Increase in heart disease alongside persistent infectious diseases.
c. Local initiatives :
  - Community programmes and low-cost innovations adapted to the region.

4. Asia
a. Diversity of healthcare systems :
  - From fully public to largely privatised systems, depending on the country.
b. Heart disease and lifestyle :
  - Rapid urbanisation, changes in diet and an increase in heart disease.
c. Traditional medicine :
  - The integration of traditional Asian medicine in prevention and treatment.

5. Latin America
a. Growth in cardiology services :
  - Investment in medical training and technology.
b. Economic challenges :
  - Inequalities in access to healthcare as a function of economic status.
c. Prevention and education :
  - Programmes focusing on nutrition, exercise and smoking reduction.

6. Australia and Oceania
a. Advanced healthcare systems :
  - Strong medical infrastructure, particularly in Australia and New Zealand.
b. Indigenous heart diseases :
  - High rates among indigenous populations, requiring specific approaches.
c. Awareness-raising initiatives :

- Public prevention and education programmes.

Although heart disease is a global challenge, approaches to its management differ considerably between regions. By understanding these differences, healthcare professionals can learn from best practice around the world and consider international collaborations to improve the management of heart patients.

The cardiology nurse in the context of global health crises

Global health crises, such as the COVID-19 pandemic, are having a considerable impact on all areas of healthcare, including cardiology. Cardiology nurses, as essential links in cardiac care teams, play a crucial role in managing these unprecedented challenges, while ensuring the continuity of cardiac care.

1. Direct impact of seizures on heart disease
a. Consequences of viruses on the cardiovascular system :
- For example, COVID-19 can lead to cardiac complications.
b. Interruption of routine care :
- Delays in diagnosis, treatment and intervention.
c. Increased stress and anxiety :
- Potentially harmful to cardiac patients.

2. Adapting practices
a. Telemedicine and remote care :
- Using technology to monitor and consult patients.
b. Modified emergency procedures :
- Prioritisation of cases according to their seriousness and the risks associated with the pandemic.

c. Protective measures :
- Personal protective equipment, reinforced disinfection protocols.

3. Human resources management
a. Redeployment :
- Some nurses may be redeployed to intensive care units or other high-need areas.
b. Accelerated training :
- Updating skills to manage the specific complications associated with the crisis.
c. Emotional support :
- Recognition of stress and fatigue, implementation of resources for the well-being of carers.

4. Education and communication
a. Informing patients :
- On the implications of the crisis for their heart condition and care.
b. Interprofessional collaboration :
- Improved communication between cardiologists, nurses and other medical specialities for optimum care.
c. Raising public awareness :
- The importance of not neglecting cardiac symptoms despite the pandemic.

5. Lessons for the future
a. Importance of preparation :
- Establish protocols for responding rapidly to future crises.
b. Enhancing the role of the nurse :
- Recognition of their adaptability and dedication in the face of challenges.
c. Innovations in care :
- Crises stimulate the adoption of new methods of care, such as telemedicine, which can continue after the crisis.

Cardiac nurses are demonstrating remarkable resilience and adaptability in the face of the challenges imposed by global health crises. They continue to provide essential cardiac care while facing the additional challenges that these crises can present. Their role is essential in ensuring continuity of care and the safety of cardiac patients at these critical times.

Collaboration and international trade

Cardiology, like many other medical fields, benefits greatly from international collaboration and exchange. These interactions can take many forms, from joint clinical research to continuing medical education and exchanges of best practice. These collaborations offer benefits not only to healthcare professionals, but also to patients, who receive cutting-edge care based on shared knowledge and experience.

1. Joint research
a. Multicentre projects :
  • Clinical studies carried out in several countries increase the diversity of patients and reinforce the validity of the results.
b. Data pools :
  • International databases allow a broader and more in-depth analysis of the data.
c. Joint financing initiatives :
  • Several countries or organisations can jointly fund large-scale research projects.

2. Training and education
a. Exchange programmes for professionals :
  • Nurses, doctors and other professionals can train abroad to acquire new skills.

b. International conferences and seminars :
- These events bring together experts from all over the world to share the latest advances in cardiology.

c. Online courses and webinars :
- Digital technology enables knowledge to be disseminated more widely to an international audience.

3. Sharing best practice

a. Networks and professional associations :
- Organisations such as the European Society of Cardiology (ESC) encourage the sharing of guidelines and recommendations.

b. Mentoring programmes :
- Recognised experts can guide and train younger or less experienced professionals from other countries.

c. Observation visits :
- Clinicians can visit other hospitals or clinics abroad to observe and learn from their methods.

4. Technological collaboration and innovation

a. Joint development of technologies :
- Countries or institutions can work together to create cutting-edge diagnostic or therapeutic tools.

b. Licences and technology transfers :
- Facilitates access to innovations for countries that do not have the necessary technology or expertise.

c. Adapting innovations to different contexts :
- For example, adapting a high-tech cardiac device so that it can be used in low-resource regions.

5. Joint responses to global challenges

a. Emerging diseases :
- Epidemics or pandemics can have an impact on cardiac patients. A coordinated response can optimise the management of these patients.

b. Demographic challenges :
- Faced with an ageing population or the emergence of new risk factors, a collaborative approach can help develop effective prevention strategies.

c. Health and humanitarian crises :
- During natural disasters or conflicts, international collaboration can guarantee the continuity of cardiac care.

International collaboration and exchange enriches cardiology by pooling the strengths, knowledge and resources of healthcare professionals around the world. These joint efforts ensure not only constant improvements in care, but also an effective, coordinated response to global challenges.

Chapter 10:
THE IMPLICATIONS
CLIMATE CHANGE
ON HEART HEALTH

Understanding the impact of natural disasters on heart patients

Natural disasters, whether earthquakes, floods, cyclones or other major climatic events, have a profound impact on healthcare systems and, in particular, on cardiac patients. These patients, already vulnerable because of their condition, can be particularly affected by the direct and indirect effects of these events.

1. Immediate physiological effects
a. Acute stress :
   * Disaster-induced stress can cause a sudden rise in blood pressure, tachycardia and potentially a heart attack.
b. Interruption of treatment :
   * Emergency evacuations and disruption of daily routine can lead to heart medication being forgotten or stopped.
c. Exposure to the elements :
   * Patients may be exposed to cold, damp or excessive heat, which can worsen their heart conditions.

2. Disruption to healthcare systems
a. Damaged infrastructure :
   * Hospitals and clinics may be damaged or destroyed, limiting access to care.

b. Drug shortages :
- Supply chains can be disrupted, leading to shortages of essential medicines for heart patients.

c. Lack of staff :
- Healthcare professionals can be personally affected or overwhelmed by the influx of patients.

3. Long-term consequences

a. Increase in chronic stress :
- Reconstruction, displacement and personal loss can contribute to a high and constant level of stress.

b. Lifestyle changes :
- Patients may adopt less healthy eating habits or reduce their physical activity, thereby worsening their heart condition.

c. Limiting access to follow-up care :
- Prolonged damage to healthcare infrastructure can make it difficult to continue regular consultations and treatment.

4. Answers and specific preparations

a. Education and awareness :
- Cardiac patients must be informed of the increased risks in the event of a disaster and how to prepare themselves.

b. Emergency kits for patients :
- Encourage patients to have an emergency kit with medicines, prescriptions and other essential supplies.

c. Emergency protocols for healthcare professionals :
- Hospitals and clinics should have specific emergency plans for the management of cardiac patients during and after a disaster.

Although natural disasters have an impact on the whole population, cardiac patients are among the most vulnerable groups. A thorough understanding of these impacts, as well as appropriate preparation and response, are essential to minimise the risks to this population.

Promoting sustainable practices in cardiology departments

Sustainability in healthcare, particularly in cardiology, is not just about protecting the environment. It is also about ensuring that resources are used efficiently, that costs are controlled and that quality care is provided in an equitable and accessible way. Here's how sustainability can be integrated and promoted in cardiology departments.

1. Reducing the ecological footprint
a. Waste management :
   * Minimisation of medical waste, reuse and recycling of uncontaminated materials.
b. Energy savings :
   * Use of energy-efficient equipment, LED lighting and optimised ventilation and heating.
c. Sustainable purchasing :
   * A selection of ethically and ecologically manufactured medical products and equipment.

2. Optimising medical processes
a. Reducing unnecessary examinations :
   * Avoiding redundancies and promoting accurate diagnoses to reduce the number of unnecessary examinations and interventions.

b. Telecardiology :
   * Encourage remote consultations to reduce patient travel and the need for hospital resources.
c. Continuing training :
   * Ensuring that staff are regularly trained in best practice to maximise efficiency and minimise errors.

3. Promoting prevention
a. Awareness-raising programmes :

- Educating the public about healthy lifestyles to reduce the incidence of heart disease.

b. Proactive monitoring of patients at risk :
- Use remote monitoring technologies to track high-risk patients, thereby avoiding unnecessary hospitalisations.

4. Collaboration and partnerships
a. Local partnerships :
- Working with other local health services to share resources, knowledge and equipment.

b. Cardiology networks :
- Create or join national or international networks to share best practice and innovation in sustainability.

5. Technological innovation
a. Regular updating of equipment :
- Invest in modern technologies, which are often more efficient and consume less energy.

b. Medical information systems :
- Use electronic medical records to reduce paperwork, improve care coordination and avoid redundant tests.

6. Community involvement
a. Reforestation programmes :
- Since the well-being of the planet is linked to heart health (air pollution, etc.), get involved in local ecological initiatives.

b. Awareness campaigns :
- Educate the community about the environmental impact of hospitals and clinics, and the measures taken to mitigate it.

Integrating sustainable practices into cardiology departments requires a holistic approach. This ranges from reducing environmental impact to optimising medical processes, innovation and collaboration. Sustainability is not only good for the planet, it also ensures the delivery of high quality, effective care that is accessible to all.

Chapter 11:
ALTERNATIVE AND COMPLEMENTARY APPROACHES IN CARDIOLOGY

Exploration of alternative therapies such as acupuncture, meditation, etc.

The integration of complementary and alternative therapies in the field of cardiology has become a subject of growing interest. These therapies, often used to complement traditional medical treatments, aim to improve heart health, reduce stress and improve patients' quality of life. However, their effectiveness varies and research continues to evaluate their clinical usefulness.

1. Acupuncture
a. Basic principles :
   • Originating in traditional Chinese medicine, it is based on the stimulation of specific points on the body to balance the flow of energy or 'Qi'.
b. Cardiac implications :
   • Some studies suggest that acupuncture can reduce blood pressure, improve symptoms of angina pectoris and reduce the frequency of arrhythmias.
c. Precautions :
   • Always ensure that the acupuncturist is certified and trained, and inform the cardiologist of any acupuncture session planned.

2. Meditation
a. Basic principles :
   • An ancient practice based on concentration, relaxation and awareness of the present moment.

b. Cardiac implications :
- Meditation can help reduce stress and blood pressure and improve heart rate variability.

c. Common types :
- Mindfulness meditation, transcendental meditation, guided meditation.

3. Yoga

a. Basic principles :
- A combination of physical postures, breathing techniques and meditation.

b. Cardiac implications :
- Can improve flexibility and muscle strength, reduce stress and have a positive impact on cardiac risk factors such as hypertension.

c. Precautions :
- Heart patients should choose a suitable style of yoga and avoid postures that could be dangerous for them.

4. Aromatherapy

a. Basic principles :
- Use of essential oils to improve physical and emotional well-being.

b. Cardiac implications :
- Certain oils, such as lavender, can help reduce stress and anxiety, factors often linked to heart disease.

c. Precautions :
- Some oils may interact with medicines or cause allergic reactions. Always do a skin test and consult a professional.

5. Biofeedback

a. Basic principles :
- Technique that teaches how to control physiological functions using machines.

b. Cardiac implications :
- Can be used to learn how to control blood pressure, heart rate and other heart health-related functions.

c. Training :
- Patients must be trained by a certified professional.

The integration of alternative therapies can offer cardiac patients additional tools for managing their health. However, it is essential to always consult a cardiologist before introducing new therapies and to ensure that these therapies are practised safely and in a way that complements traditional medical management.

Integration of these therapies as part of an overall care plan

Modern medicine increasingly recognises the value of alternative therapies as a complement to conventional approaches, especially in the field of cardiology. Integrating these therapies into an overall care plan aims to provide holistic patient management. Here's how this could be achieved:

1. Initial assessment of the patient
Before integrating any alternative therapy:
a. **Medical assessment:** Identify the patient's current condition, medicines taken and treatments in progress.
b. **Assessment of the patient's needs and preferences:** Some patients may be more inclined to try meditation, others acupuncture, and so on.
c. **Risk-benefit assessment:** Ensuring that the introduction of an alternative therapy does not pose a risk to the patient.

2. Creation of an integrated care plan
a. **Combining treatments:** For example, a patient could have conventional drug treatment for hypertension and supplement this with acupuncture sessions.

b. Regular monitoring: regular appointments to assess the effectiveness of the integrated care plan.

c. Flexibility: Be prepared to adjust the plan if a particular approach is not working or if the patient wants to try something different.

3. Training and education

a. Informing the patient: Ensure that the patient understands why a specific therapy is recommended, its benefits and limitations.

b. Staff training: Nurses, doctors and other healthcare professionals should be trained in, or at least informed about, alternative therapies as part of the care plan.

4. Interdisciplinary collaboration

a. Integrated care team: Include specialists in alternative therapies, such as acupuncturists or meditation instructors, in the care team.

b. Regular communication: Ensure that all parties are informed of ongoing treatments, adjustments and patient reactions.

5. Assessment and monitoring

a. Measuring effectiveness: Using standardised tools to assess the impact of alternative therapies on the patient's heart health and overall well-being.

b. Patient feedback: Incorporate patient feedback to continue to personalise and improve the care plan.

c. Regular updates: Recommendations and data on alternative therapies are evolving. Ensure that the care plan remains up to date.

Integrating alternative therapies into a comprehensive cardiology care plan requires a careful, personalised and evidence-based approach. It offers the opportunity to address the patient's needs holistically, considering both the physiological and emotional aspects of heart health.

CONCLUSION

Satisfactions and challenges
of the cardiology nursing profession.

The profession of cardiology nursing is both complex and rewarding. As in many areas of healthcare, it offers its share of successes and challenges. Exploring these aspects can help future nurses prepare and fully understand what lies ahead.

Job satisfaction :
- **Positive impact on patients' lives:** Helping patients navigate their cardiac journey, whether it's prevention, treatment or rehabilitation, is extremely rewarding.
- **Teamwork:** Working closely with a multidisciplinary team (cardiologists, surgeons, other nurses, physiotherapists) offers a learning and support experience.
- **Constant developments in the field:** Cardiology is a rapidly evolving field with new research, techniques and technologies. It's exciting to be at the forefront of these innovations.
- **Continuing education: There are** always opportunities to learn, whether through training, workshops or conferences.
- **Professional recognition:** Receiving thanks from patients and their families or being recognised by your peers for your work has a positive impact on morale.

Business challenges :
- **Emotional charge:** Cardiology can involve life-and-death situations, and managing these intense moments can be emotionally difficult.

- **High workload:** Cardiac units can be very busy, with many patients requiring complex care.
- **Physical demands:** Standing for long hours, transferring patients or using heavy equipment can be physically demanding.
- **Stress: Due to** the critical nature of cardiology, there can be situations of intense stress, particularly during emergencies.
- **The need for continuous updating:** While the constant evolution of the field is exciting, it also requires professionals to keep constantly up to date.
- **Difficult communication:** Communicating serious diagnoses, managing patient expectations or dealing with worried families can be difficult.
- **Dealing with the end of life:** Even with the best care, not all patients recover. Dealing with death and the grieving process can be a trying part of the job.

Cardiology nurses play an essential role in the care of cardiac patients. Although it brings many challenges, the rewards and positive impacts it offers make it a rewarding and vital profession. The key for nurses is to find a balance, seek support when needed and continually remind themselves of the crucial importance of their role.

The importance of passion and commitment in this medical speciality.

Cardiology, like many other medical specialties, requires not only technical expertise and in-depth knowledge, but also genuine dedication and passion. Passion and commitment are essential components that can determine a healthcare professional's success, quality of patient care and personal fulfilment. Here's why these two elements are particularly crucial in the field of cardiology:

1. The Complexity of Cardiology :

Cardiology is a constantly evolving field, with new research, techniques and treatments emerging regularly. Having a passion for the specialty can motivate professionals to stay up to date and continue learning throughout their career.

2. The stakes are high:

Heart disease is one of the leading causes of death worldwide. The potential seriousness of heart disease requires professionals not only to be technically proficient, but also to have a deep commitment to each and every patient.

3. Patient Relations :

The relationship between a cardiac patient and their nurse or doctor is often a long-term one. Passion and commitment help to establish a solid relationship based on trust, which is essential for the patient's care and well-being.

4. The Emotional Impact :

Faced with often stressful situations and life-and-death decisions, a deep commitment to the profession helps professionals to navigate these difficult times while providing the best possible care.

5. Team dynamics :

Cardiology is collaborative. Working with a multidisciplinary team requires open communication and a shared dedication to patient care. Personal commitment strengthens team unity and collaboration.

6. Medical Ethics :
Passion and commitment reinforce medical ethics, ensuring that every decision is taken in the best interests of the patient.

7. Job satisfaction :
Passion for the job fuels daily motivation, providing greater job satisfaction despite the challenges encountered.

In cardiology, as in many other medical fields, technique and knowledge are fundamental. However, without passion and commitment, it is difficult to achieve excellence, establish deep bonds with patients or stay motivated in the face of constant challenges. These intangible qualities are often the pillars that sustain healthcare professionals throughout their careers, helping them to make a significant difference to the lives of their patients.

GLOSSARY OF MEDICAL TERMS.

A glossary of medical terms in cardiology would be a valuable addition for readers, particularly those who are new to the field. The following is a non-exhaustive list of some common medical terms in cardiology and their definitions:

- **Arrhythmia:** Disturbance of the normal heart rhythm, whether too fast, too slow or irregular.
- **Angiography:** X-ray examination of the arteries after injection of a contrast product to visualise possible obstructions or anomalies.
- **Angioplasty:** technique used to dilate a blocked artery using a balloon.
- **Anticoagulant :** Drug that prevents blood clotting, thereby reducing the risk of thrombosis.
- **Atherosclerosis:** thickening and hardening of the arteries due to the formation of atheromatous plaques (fatty deposits).
- **Cardiomyopathy: A** disease of the heart muscle that affects the heart's ability to pump blood.
- **Defibrillator:** Device used to administer an electric shock to the heart in order to restore a normal heart rhythm.
- **ECG (Electrocardiogram) :** Recording of the electrical activity of the heart.
- **Echocardiography:** Imaging technique that uses ultrasound to visualise the structure and function of the heart.
- **Endocarditis:** Inflammation of the inner lining of the heart, often due to infection.
- **Hypertension:** Abnormally high blood pressure.

- **Infarction:** necrosis of part of the heart muscle due to a lack of oxygen supply, generally caused by a blockage in a coronary artery.
- **Ischaemia:** Reduction or cessation of blood flow to a part of the body, often due to arterial obstruction.
- **Myocardium:** Heart muscle.
- **Pericardium:** Membrane surrounding the heart.
- **Stent :** Small tubular device used to keep an artery open after angioplasty.
- **Valvulopathy:** Disease affecting one or more of the heart valves.
- **Vasodilator:** Drug which dilates blood vessels, thereby increasing blood flow.
- **Ventricle:** One of the two large chambers of the heart that expels blood into the circulation.

This glossary is only an introduction to the many terms used in cardiology. For a book intended to be a comprehensive reference on the subject, a more exhaustive list would be necessary, covering a wider range of terms, including those relating to new technologies and recent advances in the field.

ADDITIONAL RESOURCES : BOOKS, WEBSITES, PROFESSIONAL ASSOCIATIONS.

Books :
- **"Cardiology for Dummies"**: An accessible guide for novices wishing to understand the basics of cardiology.
- **"Oxford Handbook of Cardiology**: A concise textbook covering most heart problems.
- **"Manual of cardiology care"**: specifically targeted at healthcare professionals and covering current care practices in cardiology.

Websites :
- American College of Cardiology (ACC): www.acc.org
  - A world-renowned site offering resources, guidelines and news on cardiology.
- European Society of Cardiology (ESC): www.escardio.org
  - A professional organisation offering resources, conferences and news for cardiologists in Europe.
- **CardioSmart** : www.cardiosmart.org
  - A site managed by the ACC, offering information to patients on heart disease and its management.

Professional associations :
- **Société Française de Cardiologie (SFC)**: For French professionals, the SFC offers resources, conferences and continuing education opportunities in cardiology.
- **Canadian Cardiovascular Society (CCS)**: The national organization for cardiologists in Canada.
- **The Cardiac Society of Australia and New Zealand (CSANZ)**: The leading organisation for

cardiology professionals in Australia and New Zealand.
- **International Society of Cardiology (ISC)**: A worldwide organisation dedicated to promoting knowledge and care in the field of cardiology.

These resources represent just a sample of the many available. I would strongly advise you to seek out and find local or region-specific resources, and to check regularly for updates and new publications.

www.ingramcontent.com/pod-product-compliance
Lightning Source LLC
Chambersburg PA
CBHW062354290526
45794CB00005B/2218